MW01225532

Hunter, Gatherer

Hunter, Gatherer

Andrea Sheldon

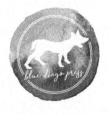

Blue Dingo Press

First Published, 2018 by
Blue Dingo Press
7 Short St, Dongara
WA Australia 6525

www.bluedingopress.com

10 9 8 7 6 5 4 3 2 1

National Library of Australia
Cataloguing-in-Publication entry available

Paperback ISBN: 978-0-6481691-0-9

Cover image and all illustrations by Andrea Sheldon

Cover design and typesetting by Chantelle Malone

Printed by Ingram Content Group LLC;
Lightning Source Australia PTY LTD

www.andreasheldon.org

For my brother.

hunting for meaning
through the cracks
in the darkness
gathering light

furniture

in my book
Women will not be
poorly upholstered furniture
nor will the men

hunting + gathering

none of us knows
what we're doing
with our lives
you'll search for meaning
for purpose
and when you get to be fifty
you'll be searching still,
and when you get to be
sixty-four and you still
don't know, you'll realise
exactly what you are
doing
with your life
what you've always been
doing
    hunting
           +
        gathering

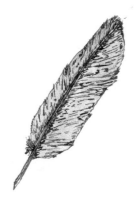

I want

I want you
to see me
I want to
show you
everything inside
and not hide
I want you
to know me
my filth,
my beauty
I want you
to devour me

taste

I'd give you my insides
if you'd have them
I'd dismantle myself
and offer you me
piece by piece
feeding you while
telling the story
of how I came
to taste this way
it's best to take
a whole mouthful
so you can experience
the full body
of flavours

the hunt

remembering
the hunt
like faint stains
on an old shirt
she'll collect
her lovers
each one
marks her
in a new way

in my mind

walking the line
between
something
and something else
to hear his voice
sharp
raw
humorous
sincere
sending shivers through
my soul
he speaks the blues
wild raving lunacy
I have to find my beat
write to keep him alive
my lover lives in my mind

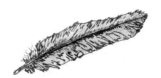

lost and found

for a long time
I couldn't find my home
lost until I realised
home is where my feet are
I'm there already

holy design

I create worlds
with words
I am humbled
by divine ingenuity
when I
and the universe
are one

384,400

looking out at the moon
it is far away tonight
small yet so large I can see it
from 384,400 kilometres away
where it sits in space and time
where it floats in the black
and if I squint I can squish it
between my thumb and forefinger
and I picture our solar system
our galaxy and universe
and am amazed at my own
expansiveness

weeds

bursting forth
from just beneath
I am that seed
germinating
deep deep deep
within
evolving emerging
larger than life
smaller than an atom

hello

to the girl that sounds
like a flower opening up
to the morning sun
when she says hello

naked sixteen

they said she was inappropriate
her nakedness offensive
her rawness precocious
they said they could
not in good taste publish
such a vulgar piece
they said her work wasn't art
they returned her self-portrait
folded in on herself crumpled
they tried to censor her
to edit her for decency
to stifle her creativity
her femininity
after all, how dare she?

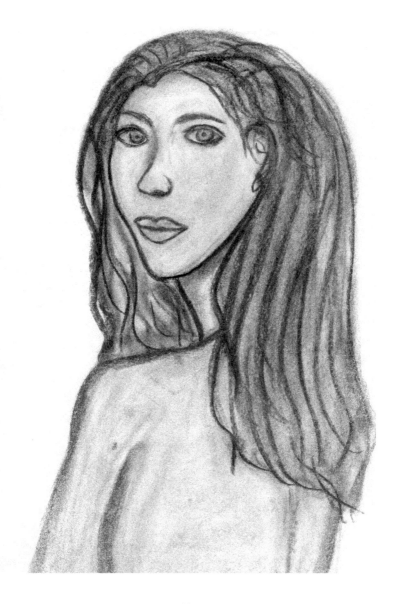

I bleed

my belly aches
it swells
I bleed
life
to give

consent

I allow myself
    the freedom
of wilderness
I feel powerful
    sexual
        woman
I own the moment
    my situation

I allow myself
    the freedom
       to play
I feel unrestrained
    childlike
        woman
ignoring should
    or shouldn't

streams

who do you run to
uninhibited, raw
being turned inside out
vulnerable when
everyone you've ever loved
has passed before your life
the dead live
bleeding solitude
sol sole soul soleil
brighten my vast night
there must be truth
within that jest
of darkness inside
where I apparently reside
though I can't say
I've experienced
anything
least of all
the bowery blues
my wounds have
been self-inflicted.
that was a lie
see, do you see?

I lie
about all I've seen
somehow I can form
no poetry
to do justice
to where I've been
I can tell you how I feel
the physicality of
my grief in the weight
of your caress
maybe you feel it too
as you dry my eyes
of the shadowed tears
life teaches us to suppress

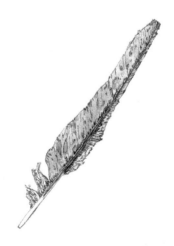

scent

the hint of a scent
on the breeze
and she's reeling
through images
long forgotten
a chill runs from
the base of her spine
like electricity
something that beckons
the scent reminds
her body of its own
corporeality.
her ribs hold her heart
like a cage
and that scent opens the door

just so

earth salt sand
ocean sweat mildew
grass dandelion
allspice fennel
and cinnamon
cardamom
warm milk & honey
burnt matchsticks
countryside
mountains forest
autumn
peppercorn
all these things
and he smells just so

the poet

the poet looked up from
her restless bus-ride kip
had she been drooling?
did anybody see?
as the brief self-conscious
semi-awareness came and
went, her eyes opened
to the stories she'd so rudely
been too self-absorbed to notice.
admonishing herself, she made
a point to engage in
the breathtaking view
from an open heart
and she lost her breath.

to her right, a heavyset
woman in her fifties
with deep brown eyes and
a nomad's heart
dressed in clothes that imply
she's let herself go, always
caring for somebody else.
she spends this time engrossed
in a dime-store romance.
looking up

            look-up!
her thoughts move
from the tingle
in the base of her spine
to the knot in her stomach
and the wretch in her heart.
for a moment she's removed
from her erotic
early morning escapade
she bleeds into herself
eyebrows raised
blinking once
            blinking twice
a nod, assured.
eyebrows crinkle
a shrug.
thin lips press
tightly in consternation
returning from her brief moment
of internal fiction
to the realism of
her harlequin.
the kind of romance
she's saved herself for

maybe things might
have been different
had she seen the horizon
from the bridge
like the poet when
she looked up
and out of herself
to the light flutter of wings
through the thick midsummer
morning haze off the river
through lines of trees
a sea-way canal gives birth
to a small vessel
she wishes
she was the bird
she wishes
she was a tug boat
she wishes

escape myself

my body tense
with untamed emotion
tearing at the seams
to escape
my gaze steady
cool
collecting information
in an attempt to ease
me out of myself
my mind racing
blind erratic
direct with uncertainty

complications

by giving in to
these rationalisations
you will never discover
what you could really do
if you simply committed
to yourself

when it is so simple, it all seems so complicated

in between

it wasn't him or her
he or she
that meant anything much
or much of anything
for any great amount
of time
it was an idea of
something mad for life
brought to a brief semi-reality
only half existing, half truth
like standing in a doorway
somewhere between
here and there, hoping.
one cannot stand still
belonging in between
hoping for very long

from inside

long awaiting
inspiration
from above
from below
from outside
ignite me
set the spark
somehow
on my own
from inside
I've caught up

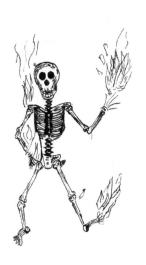

shadow selves

I want to share with you
myself
what exists in the deep
recesses of my heart
what exists in hiding
I think that's what
scares you
intrigues you

muse

I keep my mind
on you
for the unattainable
for what exists
only inside of me
you brought it out
what's mine
the passion, the poetry
but when you left
I stumbled wounded
my freedom caved
in upon itself
collapsed
I keep you
inside of me
to keep myself
and am constantly reminded
that you were never you
but a reflection of me

photographs

images imprisoned in time
time imprisoned in images
trapping the soul
my soul scattered into
thousands of photographs
my shadow has an echo
I have no shadow, only an echo
a memory of a shadow
held hostage in a snapshot

I stand alone

standing outside
your circle of friends
causes no discomfort to me
I'm starving for something
you can't feed me
it isn't your responsibility
I'm standing outside
laughing and
dancing alone

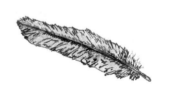

loner

they'll watch you
wander on, fascinated
baffled by your solitude
because they see a lonely
wasteland where you find
a whole world in the wilds
a freedom you know like
the back of your hand, and
that is why they could never
share it with you

whole self

I felt too reticent
        and uneasy
                to let myself
                        out
what you saw
        were glimpses
I am afraid
           if you could see
              my entirety
                  your fear
                        would get the better
                              of you

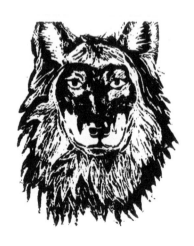

your song

the song you sing
when you aren't listening
rings solitude
right through my being
your waking words
conceal
what your deeper worlds
fight to explain

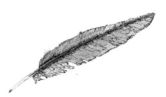

if, I am

if I am
withholding
I am dishonest
with myself

if I am
forthcoming
I am too intense
for you

fear of heights

when you've hit the
ground face first
before you've ever
jumped
standing at the top
looking down

terrified of
a free fall
to the bottom
SPLAT

can you truly
appreciate the beauty
from above
in fear?

brick wall

as we dive deep
into each other's eyes
I see you peeking out
over your brick wall
painted with dreams
I recognise it immediately
I have one too
I reach up
onto the tips
of my toes hoping
someday you'll invite me
to the other side
sometimes I see you try

stone wild heart

I lament my love
falling
to a desolate landscape
yet it persists
in the face of drought
I wait for him with
his stone heart
and his wild shadow
I could let another hold me
a simple act
the contact consoles me
though all I want is
that stone wild heart

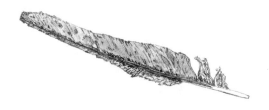

hunted

those eyes
      seeping
         into
           through
             around
               enveloping
                 consuming
                   me

remembering

I keep coming back
to your eyes, those eyes
as they touch mine
burning deep poetry

I return to your fingertips
and your hands as they explore
travelling landscapes
of my desire

remembering your words
your laughter your soft reply
your breath tickles my ear
as you sleep

we walked

I took the route
we walked together
it made me feel
closer to
you

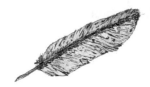

lost

he asks if I'm lost
I answer always
and never

love is a wanderer

I knew that he loved me
in that moment
if never again
but that moment
was all that existed
until the motions
of energy
changed direction
with the wind

daydreaming

clarity of your wisdom
daydreaming my way
into or out of
layers of existence
in our cave

our own little world
and he was lost
in the music
in the black

and then
I was
outside
walking the desert
under a setting sun

ode to

losing the one
true love I never had
I mourn his demise
aware it was my own
it sucked me in
and never spit me out
had I lost my mind
or found myself?
child why do you cry?
I weep for a loss I have
no memory of, I weep
for you my love

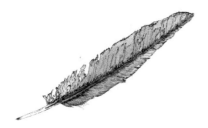

illumination

we flew together
the four of us
over the clouds
second star to the right
and straight on till morning
effortless and in love
with life
        with each other
every touch lived
to the fullest
and with all the meaning
in the world
expanded
        expanding
with our hearts
creating and consuming
and on and on
        all lives
past the perception of death
        eternal life
we sang together
we sang
the song of the universe

shadows

wild nights
have faded
into long summer days

a creature of shadows
basking in sunlight
forgets the gentle kiss
of the moon

a fallen star
stumbles through
blinding light
without the darkness
to guide her way

the creature of shadows
climbing the death trail
whistles a familiar tune

the fallen star
searching for her kin
hears the echo of
a song on a distant breeze

now

time speeding
beyond the moment
live in the now
but it's already past

bodhisattva

when I was a child
I dreamed of being a bodhisattva
where did that dream go?
I was born a teacher
and learned to become a student

restless

restless
for something more
something unknown
somewhere unexplored
I forget to mind my
surroundings

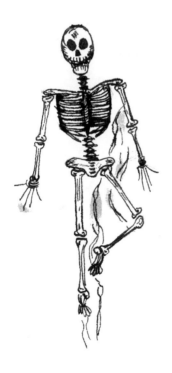

ink water

they flew in a line
the wind whistling
        through their wings
                in the night
calling out in rank
a vague honking song
lights the silence of the dark

as the bats swoop
        and flutter
                yes they flutter
over the still ink water
listening to the sound
of their flight echo against
the gentle heave of the lake
searching for bugs to eat

the sun has long set
the breeze
makes ripples through
the water
sparkling in the light
of the moon

revolve

each line
a message from god
if only you could read
the leaves and the grass
like brail
with their sunburnt tips
they fight to maintain
their living colours

in the winter
it rains green
the ravens rejoice
flame ravaged earth
sighs relief.

the glass is always
half empty come summer
in the red dust swirling
into hungry sparks
ready to consume again.

her smile

she smiles bright
softening the bumps
the taunts
the blows
her smile
opens a crack in my heart
her smile
invites a little sunlight in

he gives pause

his gentle smile
makes her heart
breathe
for a moment
inspire, expire
there is no space
between
he'll never know
the light he brings

so much more

I come here
to contemplate
beauty
and fall in love
with myself again
the tides bind me
to you
the stars guide me
through.
the sandy earth
under my feet
reminds me,
there's so much more
to know
and I want, need, long
to know

salt

she doesn't stay
to be a part of anything really
but to be apart.
to listen, see, feel, taste, smell

the sound he plays
creeps up her spine
like a serpent
in a death embrace
it becomes entwined

where it vibrates
and the sound of her joy
becomes something to
see, taste, feel

his sound becomes the
salt on her lips

foxhole

when she hides
he watches her go
his fear is her fear
her shadow realm, her foxhole
he's found her secrets
he soothes her pain
the illusion is that he has
healed her with his love

displaced

displaced
I feel winter in my bones
I wake cold, shivering
under blankets piled to the ceiling
the weight of them grounds me
to return to dreaming
there's no place like home
but my slippers aren't rubies
and the road is red dust
the ravens follow me
call to me, "you are
home, home, home."

but it is summer, not the winter
my bones tell me it should be
and the sun beats my shoulders
with a kiss as my bare feet
meet the scorched earth
I don't sink into its depths
the earth is hard and dry
and I've forgotten the sharp bite
of frost and the feeling of snow flakes
melting as they land soft on my skin

In this place, I am other
a foreign object that never quite settles
inside, I am an entire landscape
covered in sweat, dirt, tears
forests, fur, and feathers
inside, I am warm
even in the cold
I am home

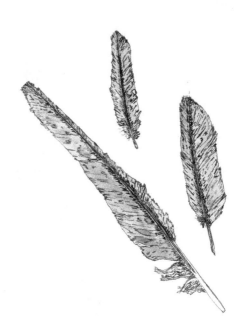

walk lightly

the pavement burns
under my toes
ouch
like matchsticks
igniting
a reminder to walk
lightly on the earth

the flames rise up
engulf me
I burn and am
reduced to cinders

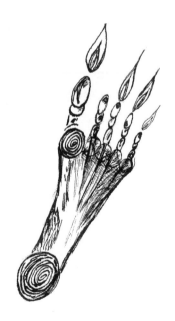

eternal and insubstantial

death occupies my mind
my mind like my body
occupies time and space
is alive, capable of exploding

I live in both life and death
in between
expiration and animation
I am a torrent raging inside
grave
devouring being devoured
eternal and insubstantial
strikingly inconspicuous
barely present
clashing states of being
breathing bereavement
in ambivalence

artful idleness

tick tick tick
the seconds lead to minutes
leading to hours of idleness
nothing stirs

her mind
engaged as it is
feels vacant
nothing moves
and time slows until
even the crisp air stands still

the sound of traffic
passing on the back road
seems to blend
with the babble of the creek

movement
the sound of that forward rush
reminds her that time will
progress with or without her

perhaps this stillness is a good thing
perhaps it affords her the luxury
of observing life as it moves
watching the clothes drying on the line
and somehow finding meaning in it

should she embrace this idleness
become still, she might
find from within herself
a whole world stirring

travelling

how are all things
         living in all things
                moving through all things
as her body dropped
         her spirit soared
                passing through to bliss
a violent awakening
         numb
chaotic torrents of rage
         build up
                ebb & flow
her spirit drops

migraine

everything is
too bright
too sharp
too loud
too piercing
everything moves
too fast
too slow
too abrupt
too aggressive
too floaty
too passive
it is all
too much
I am
disoriented
disembodied
the patterns
of the tiles in the floor
don't help

growing up

years of nightly terrors
something sinister
trying to grab hold
to possess me

sometimes it is invisible
a looming presence
and I sense it and flee

mostly, though, it takes
the form of an old woman
or a little girl sitting next to me
on a bus or in a cafe

she engages with me, sweetly
at first and often it takes time
for me to recognise it, but I do

breathless, I whisper, "it's you"
she replies with a searing silence
and a harrowing smile
as she reaches for me

I try to flee but she catches up
quickly and grabs hold
I become heavy, torpid, paralysed
I'm suffocating

sometimes before I wake
I can feel her seeping
into my lungs
trying to take control

I'm fighting, screaming
"get out!" my voice changes
becomes not mine "get out!"
I wake up

when I was a little girl,
I dreamed I could fly
all I had to do was jump
and believe

I would float up, up, up
and I would be free
soon I was teaching others
how to fly too
it is what I came here to do

at some point I stopped
flying and started to flee
hitting the ground running
from this shadowed presence
I can't actually see

but I know it wants to take control
to make me heavy
under the weight of its gravity
and all I want to do
is fly again

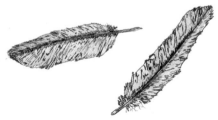

erode

she feels dry
brittle
stuck
in an emotion
she can't physically express
trapped inside unidentifiable
discontent
she can't place her finger on
how does one locate and fix
something so elusive
it might not exist
it exists
she knows it exists
because she hears it
moving around in the walls
in her very foundation
eroding her
she hears it
whispering as she dreams
she doesn't feel quite herself
her skin doesn't fit
her brain malfunctions
she fears a slip into delirium
but the view
from that thin line
when the moon is high
is so beautiful
she's awestruck

being human

in a constant state of becoming
something different
always the same
change is the only consistency
in life entangled
in the inevitability of death
acceptance becomes freedom
we feed ourselves to flee
our food becomes our poison
the sustenance we crave
cannot sustain us
we become a daily cycle
of nourishing ourselves
on our own destruction
the very nature of man
in constant seeking
blinded by the search
he never finds
what he's looking for
but he'll destroy us all to get there

wallpaper

blurred in the background
I'm out of focus
he's the star of this picture
you can tell by the outline of his jaw
he doesn't even realise
I've faded
I've blended into
the wallpaper
it was only a matter of time
no one suspects
the wallpaper
people will say anything when
they think nobody is listening
wallpaper carries secrets
like whispers in trees
even the hideous
pearlescent floral kind
I can tell you a story about
life, death, and the journey between
you won't hear me though
I'm out of focus
blurred in the background

blinded

blinded
by his hunger
I am his meat
a flesh to eat
a warm body
to sustain him

amor vincit omnia

he'll take her body
and call it her soul
when his notes
belong to her pleasure
but he's playing an empty vessel
filling her with his hopes
his dreams, his expectations
he empties himself into her
until she has grown fat
with his self-deceptions and
his heart grows heavy
under her weight
so he casts her off
to escape himself

fickle

he tells me
I am his
pumpkin patch
he has a new
nickname
for me
every single day

push

when push comes
to shove
he stands
in the middle
watching me
what's he waiting for?
he likes the effect
he has
he consumes me
to feed his emptiness

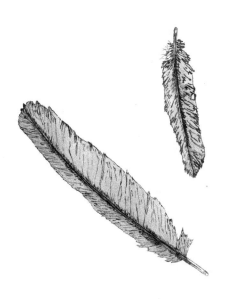

grey

I live in shadows
of my own emotions
          in between
                    grey
he whispers in my ear
soft violence
I can't see him
I can't see myself

that day

when she woke up, she
was covered in bruises
up her arms and neck

she undressed
and as she stepped into
the shower to wash
him off of her
she saw her reflection
from behind
scrapes and bruises down
her slender back

clumps of blood
from where her hair
had been ripped out
diluted in the water
pooling at her feet
the pain pulsing through
her body ached
with a numbing shame

she dried herself
slow, deliberate
she walked naked
into the living room
to the couch
where he slept

his eyes
filled with tears
hers with rage
"if you ever hurt me again"
through her bruised throat
she could only manage
a whisper
"I'll have you arrested
I will press charges
you won't just lose
me
you will lose
everything"

"I love you"
he said
"I'm sorry"
she couldn't let him see
the tears
she walked away
she got dressed
she covered up
she left for work

she lost a piece
of herself keeping
his secret as if
it was her own shame

a choice that stole
her voice
inflicting wounds
deeper than his brutality
scar tissue that lingered
long after he was gone

outside

his heart breaks as he looks outside
for the answers hidden within
and he sighs to ease the pain
that does not end

she left

if you ever leave me
no-one will take me in
I'll be the tramp
from beauty and the beast
he says to her, lips stained
red burgundy

you taught me

physical violence
as a gesture
of friendship
kinship
love

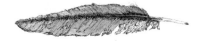

creeping

there's a spider
crawling up your thigh
anxious
to deposit
its sweet venom

dirty talk

I saw a man
on the train today
he was staring
conspicuously
at a girl's chest
when he started
talking dirty
to her
she pretended
he wasn't there
and as he continued
his onslaught
I began to think
he was a figment
of my imagination

beauty in suffering

how do you find the beauty
        in such things
                in such pain
                        in such ugliness
there must be some meaning
        some secret
                to bearing
                        the suffering

spirit endures

spirit endures
more than you know
surviving all the bullshit
is an act of rebellion
as you shed the you
you no longer need
and become whole again

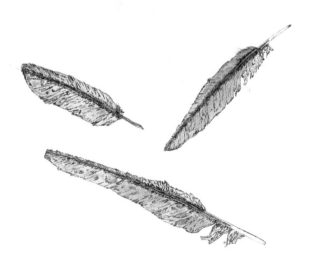

the wrong way

fly away
to where? from what?
you're my excuse for being here
I forgot to live
I learned to love
the wrong way
I learned to be loved
as a possession
occupied and held
stop

contrarily

his enveloping arms
soothed her once
now bind her
in silk ribbons
and any resistance
strengthens the restraints
fighting to take flight
screaming, laughing
contrarily
she hides
in a hole
in a corner
in a closet
buried within
quiet
she dreams of rapture
but finds silence

soulmates

lovers entangled
drawing blood
along the lines of
codependency
ensuring mutual
destruction.
strangled but
they've only ever
known this kind of
love

gone

trapped inside your box
of lovers
and letters
I can't change

what's been locked
away
but you don't see
what I won't say
you'd listen
but you wouldn't
hear me anyway

your thoughts are too
loud for me
to breathe
your love is too
proud for me
to leave
but I'm already
gone
don't you see?

not yours

I am not
yours
to judge
to give value
to devalue
with each passing
expectation disappointed
your ideas are yours
they do not touch
me
you have no right
to my mind
nor my body
I am not yours
this home is mine

hidden deep

what it is to sit, waiting
for inspiration
to express eloquently
what is hidden in the deep
recesses of the soul
words fall short

incomplete

I don't know
who I am
I can't hear
my voice
I'm on display
in a glass box
and I can't see
what they see
I can see
my hands
my hands feel
everything it is
I want to say but
they can't seem to
create
they hunger
but can't taste
the scent of
inspiration
hangs heavy
in the air

it lingers
silently mocking
we are all
incomplete
racing headlong
blind
thirsty for meaning
but when you
write it down
it disappears

danse macabre

not for anyone
not for rhythm
nor sex
their bodies move
against the music
unaware
Dionysus whispers
through their hips
absent noises
move from their lips
back and forth
through absent ears
but their bodies know

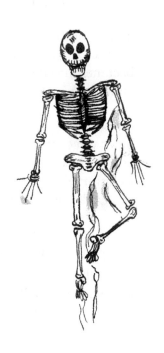

falsehoods

paradise is lost on those who are
so easily deceived
when knowledge once found
bears weight, responsibility

a deeper understanding
of the way things work
there is a choice to make
turn away to assimilate
to what is socially acceptable
to be well adjusted

false fronts bring joy
to false eyes and when authenticity
becomes the latest platitude
another word lost to pretence

it is so easy to stop hearing your
inner voice over the voice you use
and the face in the mirror becomes
so distorted by the faces you wear
you can't remember what's genuine, who's true

the only way out is through
the space the silence takes to
listen more deeply and stop
playing at being human

marionette

she understands now
the antagonist of her nightmares
symbols she mistook caught her breath
and held it hostage, taciturn
turning her body into a puppet
a dancing marionette
her performances wooden
smile pretty
keep dancing
keep smiling
and when she bleeds
she's a cotton stuffed doll
good for a squeeze
an example of expert taxidermy
looking for signs of life
a mountain of cotton and dried blood
because even on her best behaviour
she leaks
climbing the mountain
to loosen the strings
she chews her way through
with her little chiclet teeth
risking a tumble to be free
and without any bindings
she's singing, dancing, bleeding, thinking
all by herself

unbound

alone
not hiding
seeking
opening doors
finding walls
searching for windows
crawling
catlike
singing at the top of my lungs
intensity unbound

threat of the fall

freedom of existence
existence of freedom
never the sum
of their perceptions
separated through
the relief of rejection
he called her out
beyond her fenced edge
she didn't realise
the threat of the fall
was an illusion
she's got nine lives

platitudes

she longs for - not more
as that might suggest that
life is measurable, that
happiness is quantifiable and
what are the parameters anyway?
but, she wants something other
she wants rapture
she doesn't know what she wants really
only, she is certain of what she doesn't
want, what she just won't do

she abhors all banalities
which brings to question
whether this is part of her
conditioning, in the same way that
others have been reared to want what
she views as trite

and an older more experienced
version of herself might
hear her diatribe and roll her eyes
at her own naive idealism
apparently she is just going through
a phase

a cliché rebellion against
the status quo, with its own brand
of platitudes, we all outgrow

will she someday fall out
of lust with life
will her ardour become memory
hidden under an overpriced haircut
will she sit down at a desk
in overpriced clothes made in
a sweatshop for under a dollar

will she someday soon be wed
in white tulle in a church with six
bridesmaids and a blushing groom
a binding legal contract to
engage in the act, to disseminate
future generations nurtured
to keep the machine running
we are after all social animals

will she bear offspring to fill
the space in her heart
with joy and meaning

because hormones
told her brain it's time
to create more of herself

will she give them proper
names and send them off to
school - an assembly line
to churn, knead and roll
the soft plump dough
to cut into generic shapes
put them into the oven to bake
with sprinkles of sugar and spice

and when the timer sounds
deviants discarded, they fall
through the cracks, but
the beautiful shapes of golden
brown sit down at a desk
in overpriced clothes made
in a sweatshop for under a dollar
there are of course, exceptions
to the rule

united

we all love
we all dream
we all hope

we all crave
we all starve
we all fade

but never together
never truly united
do we stand

collective

yet another interruption in
my peculiarity
the collective conscious
washes over me, bleaching out stains
sparkling whites, and sun kissed hues
snuffing out any flicker of self
hope I hold in my dreams
when I am broken and beaten
a malleable mass like a sponge
soaking up fallacies like gospel
truths, a propagandist's
dream verisimilitude
a population anaesthetized
into submissive participation
by how truth-like it all is and
my dissentious idealism seems more
like delusion silently skipping stones
into the waves of collective delirium

greed

strength or hindering action
feeding the megalomania
that feeds the nation
when hope is in a nation
that starves its hungry
to satiate its greed
        getting fat on your flesh
picking its teeth with your bones
hope is quietly dissipating

chess

I can't play chess
I have no mind for war
I care too much
for the lives of my pawns

they become
animated
with souls, lives, stories
they become
indispensable friends
I refuse to be
the kind of queen
who would sacrifice
her subjects
and call it collateral

forsaken

we've searched for God
everywhere but here
we've created heaven and hell
in the likeness of man
God hid in plain sight
reaching out through our hearts
where nobody bothered to look
while screaming obscenities, forsaken.

so-called free

being
in the centre
of a vast open field
with a roof over my head
finding nothing
in any direction
not even the sky

becoming lost

I'd love to live
in my own delirium
though I fear
becoming
lost

leaden

higher than rooftops
I sit leaden
in the weight
of my senses
looking down I watch
as they fly weightless
free of intellectual unrest
my emotions contradict
my freedom

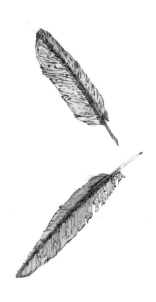

teddy bear picnic

there's a little imposter
in us all
a feigned expertise
sometimes I am afraid
of when the jig is up
when they'll figure
me out
my intelligence
my creative intrigue
my adult clothes
will be stripped away
and I'll be left
standing
seven years old
in the middle of
a teddy bear picnic

tiger lily

tiger lilies again
this time she stops to smell them
a light sweetness that leaves
her nose covered in pollen
the colour of dried blood

she never picks flowers
she thinks it's barbaric
they're much too beautiful
to cut their lives short
for her vanity

but she picks one anyway
to carry with her
to remind herself
of who she is
and where she's going

subterranean

subterranean lovesick blues
stolen moments in borrowed time
everyone has secrets
everyone lies to themselves
if only for a short while
but when those moments
honour a personal truth
loyal only to the heart
what's secret is kept secret
as an expression
of the gilded self
an act of rebellion
an act of self-preservation

cavernous

did he get out alive?
did she survive the night?
with a secret
there is no right
he looks at her with new eyes
and she sees the stars
creating a cave
their sacred space
he runs his fingers
along blood's memory
without judgement
extending his thirst
for understanding
an unfamiliar sentiment
building blocks of an apology
for breaking her heart
he need only gather pebbles
forgiveness came to him
without his asking

when you're gone

joggers marching
in unison
under a hazy sun
to a new kind of
dictatorship

drunk boys
at a bar
discussing the joys
of foreskin
under the dizzy moon
animated

too many pages
spent not wasted
on the lack of you
even in your presence
but we're together
as we dream
when you're gone

hold fast

hold fast
of memories
half faithful to
the reality of things
a contagious romanticism
always sweeter as epithets
afterthought will be the death
of us all
running from passion
present moment
love
life in remembrance

gotcha

he pushed
she fell
he caught hold
she fell into him
he held tight
she fell in love
he turned away
to look back
over his shoulder
smile and wink
gotcha

keep me

I wanted to love you
not to keep you
I think you fear
wanting to keep me

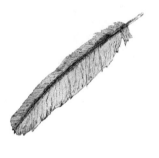

narcissus

earnest turned frivolous
concluded evening overlooks
my eyes a mirror
reflecting light and shape
or lack of

do I
cause you discomfort?
does the sight
of yourself
excite you?

full mind closed eyes

what are you trying to hold?
what idea do I represent?
what fantasy am I?
what role do I play?
it isn't me
your mind is full
but your eyes are closed

the perfect fort

losing my footing
keeping your pace
I had a dream last night
I saw you as I slept

building up
the perfect fort
made of pillows

our own little stronghold
and we were safe
for a moment, hidden
from the world

but then you
tore it down
with me inside
laughing
        joyful
        afraid
        menacing

only to build it
right back up again
is it a game you enjoy?

self preservation

you open up your wounds
to show me how you bleed
trying to convince yourself
how deep you run and then hide
when I show you mine
but please don't be surprised
upon your return if you find
me sweetly aloof here and
there and gone already
yours is a depth that needs
an audience, but your martyr
performance leaves much
to be desired.

the things I've seen

when my eyes aren't windows
but mirrors
and when you look into them
I reflect the parts of yourself
you wish you could hide
from what you'd rather not see
there is no forgetting
it cannot be unseen
I always thought you had to
be honest with yourself
to traverse your own depths
your own contradictions
in order to evolve.
maybe I was wrong
maybe all you need to do is
avoid mirrors

longing

and off it goes
my mind racing
to keep up
what am I
holding onto?

a near tangible illusion
an idea
I've built you up
my longing a mirage
of what I most desire

you feed my chaos
and I bleed for you
at any cost to my self
I've fallen on dark days

you were so unfamiliar
in all the familiar ways
I recognised in you
my own creative power
and I loved you for it

but all the passion
in the world couldn't
satisfy such a longing
and I grew bored
    of you

his silence

his silence
sucks me in
standing naked
in the centre
of an empty room
filled with words
spoken
left unspoken
and pitch black

subtleties of self-doubt

subtle clues
to my bitter sweet
end
become loud, clear
I melt under the sun
and am washed away
when it rains through May
if only I could speak clearly
if only he could hear me
but when I think he speaks
the same language
it is not he
but my own self-doubt
which leaves me frozen
come December

you rushed through

you rushed through
you didn't see me
as soon as you were inside
it was like I wasn't there

high adventure

your high adventure
is my downfall
I speak of nothing
when I tell you my dreams
would it hurt you terribly
to dream with me

hidden self

the one place she experienced
freedom
she's hidden her soul
from the world, from herself
and she's forgotten why

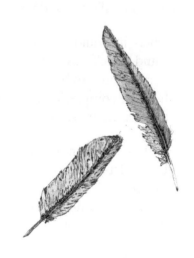

hush

melancholia seeps
into places it doesn't belong
I find my anger suffocated
the flames diminished by
the claustrophobic damp
comfort of that internal violence
where a woman quells her rage
into the safety of sadness

where it should be empowering
I find myself cowering to give myself
permission – to be hard
because compassion and anger
are not mutually exclusive

in dreams I own my anger
I don't let sadness overcome
the multiplicity of my feeling
I don't let sadness overtake
the discomfort of my rage

instead of getting lost down
the rabbit-hole of anger
internalized into sadness
I get angry and then
do something about it

torpefy

one by one
they slip away
they lose their grip
I watch them go
helpless
as they forget
their own power
voluntarily sedated
the world becomes
medicated
they lost God
and found numbness
in an escape from
the heavy realism
of their lives

unknown sickness

there is something invading me
pervading my being
a heaviness
a tightening in my chest
an overwhelming sense
of un-satisfactoriness
grabbing hold of my breath
rendering me without life
or lucid thought

water

she lives with
a broken body
her legs like lead
her head full of dread
"I always knew I would
die in water"
holding her breath long
enough to hear her heart
beating
like someone trapped in
a magicians box
"but not today"

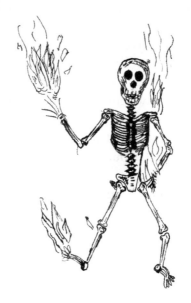

migraine II

to explain the feeling
a heightened awareness of the senses
debilitating hypersensitivity, confusion
lights fluorescent flashing
sends jolts of lightening to the back of my eyes
blinding burning aching
behind my vision
things move from crisp disembodied images
to a blur of light, colour and smell
shapes lose form to shadows

sound rumbles and shrieks through my body
a whisper assaults my throbbing brain
which pounds in unison with all the sounds
a plastic bag crumples, footsteps,
the train pulls in flashing lights
through my ears
makes my body ache, throb, groan
too loud my stomach lurches
I can't see what you're saying
the smells - putrid flesh, rotting on bones
my eyes burn
my stomach lurches

neglect

I wonder if neglected creativity
can take on a life of its own
a beautiful and grotesque creature
haunting your dreams
aching to possess you
hovering over you, whispering
in your ears as you sleep
"let me speak, I have something to say"
"why have you deserted me?"
but if you wait too long
to give and to take
she'll pack her bags and walk away
she won't look back
she has too much self respect
        to remain abandoned

resplendence

wandering through reverie
how much time does it take
to render you forever changed?
can one little thing, one moment
change your entire perception
your entire direction?
I find myself sitting under a tree
seeking relief
from the sharp midday sun
beating down on our backs
I find his face, this place
strangely familiar
as if from a dream
he sits rolling a crystal
between his thumb and forefinger
the dirt roads are paved in quartz
and he is resplendent

a kiss

here is
the end of the road
mister
is this what you want?
a kiss? mister
kiss the morning
the sun elated
celebrating life
love, death
a kiss of mourning
the feared and elusive
inevitable

pieces

I woke up
in your room alone
surrounded by your smell
surrounded by your belongings
surrounded by pieces of you
and I fell to pieces
my soul undressed
piece of armour by piece of armour
until she stood naked in
front of me
gazing at her own reflection
and she said to me
"you're beautiful when you're in love"
I scrambled
searching for the armour
but she was too quick
she took me to pieces
I'm a heap on the floor
you can scoop me up
or sweep me under the bed

your love

waiting for your love
not to be something
dangled in front of me
like a mechanical rabbit
keeps me running
keeps me racing in circles
when your love is something
I can curl up into
fall into and trust
that you'd catch me
but I keep on running
your love is within my reach
your love is withheld
I'm out of breath

ravens

she lived in a house of lies
sad, silenced and alone
she cried out from her heart
sentiments that fell on deaf ears
until the ravens came
they offered her kinship
they offered her truth
they offered her home
they sang to her - creeeeeek -
and nobody else could hear
the music in the noise
surrounded by ravens, she sat
she swayed to their poetry and
they sang her back to life
soon she was singing with them
- creeeeek - it never mattered
if nobody else could hear
the music in the noise

your spiritual debris

nails scratching
clawing
teeth clenching
biting
bodies entwined
sleepwalking
through life
I'm pummeled by
your spiritual debris
collateral damage
I have this
recurring nightmare
I'm underwater
climbing a wall
I can't float
the water
weighs me down
fills my lungs
every inch I gain
I'm dragged back
I begin to drown
nails scratching
clawing, bleeding
teeth clenching
I'm shattering

house of love

he built a home out of rotting
wood and festering lies
and wondered when it crumbled
he told her the house had new
solid foundations and steel dreams
he told her the roof would never leak
he thought she wouldn't notice the black
mould seeping through the ceiling
growing out from the corners
down the walls creeping
into her lungs with every breath
she took in this false house of love
he thought she wouldn't see the ghosts
peeking in through cracked windows
he thought it wouldn't matter as long as
she saw what he was telling her to see
as long as she suspended her disbelief
as long as they both lived in his imaginary
house of love, so she closed her eyes
and told herself she was blind

their house of love was a beautiful fiction
becoming a dark prison full
of menacing shadows, she fragmented
sick, suffocated, and afraid
day and night trapped without light
and when she stopped looking over her shoulder
in her peripheral vision the veil lifted
and she could see clearly
the ugliness she was living
so she closed her eyes tight, and tried
as hard as she might to tell herself
lie to herself, convince herself
they had a beautiful home, he built it with love
truth, though, being a persistent weed
took seed deep deep deep in her heart
the mould blackened the walls
water ran like congealed blood
the cracks in the windows the walls and the floors
opened up to the creepers and the vines
reclaiming their house of lies
and now lost and alone in the jungle that's grown
up through the cracks in the floor, she's entangled
– broken-hearted without shelter from
                                    the coming storm

you left me

you left me
terrified and alone
in the middle of a storm
and it was tearing me
apart

you left me
behind
in the middle of a storm
it tore away jagged
parts of me, frayed
and here I am
transformed

deep in the night

the rage came on
deep in the night
the line between
reality and night
terrors blurred

it became
a nocturnal ritual
a mind riddled
betrayed
burdened with grief
the loss of love
a body twisted in pain

the moon is high
only ruins

and rubble
surround the bed
where she sleeps
where he sleeps
where *they* slept

are things
as they truly are
in the world of shadow
by the light of stars?

or does the shadow
world cast darkness
where there ought to
be light - where the stars
cannot reach

trees bleed too, you know

a thick sticky sadness
carried on the wind
catches in the leaves
trickles slowly
seeping into the trees
that cry out in the night
and weep thick sticky tears
resin of their plight
their branches overhang
a crumbling house
everything held together
by a silk thread

but not soon enough

though you cut me
deep
I've removed
your knives
I'll return them to you
soon enough

these old wounds
left open for so long
now scars
fading
into the past
I'll forget you
soon enough

I saw it in my dreams

I saw it in my dreams
taking hold of my nightmares
creeping into my waking thoughts
terrorising my hopes
I begin to unravel
promises I've made
to myself seem vacant yet
so burdened I need to
empty myself of the fear
my wary heart pumps through
my veins like little threads
pulling, I'm coming apart
piece by piece
I shed yesterday
I am free

diving

diving
into the deep
blue of my own eyes

I am becoming
aware of the light
beyond my own shadow

I grow towards it
my home
no longer bound to
gathered darkness
my mind
no longer riddled
spinning, disoriented
I am free
from the prison
of my own creation

metamorphose

I've been catching fire
for so long now
charred flesh
and gathered bones
I wonder what
kind of creature
will emerge from
the flames
something magnificent

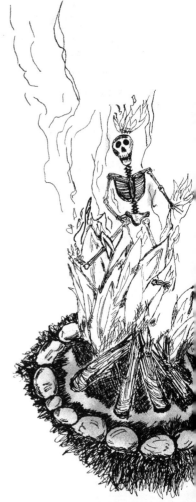

change

I accept change
to die
I am reborn
to run from it
is to stagnate

I sacrifice myself
to myself
growing
creating
evolving

myself perceives
a life far greater
than that of
who I am today

a bitch's brew

dark matter
a witch's brew
black coffee in a cup
the size of a cauldron
coffee-grind divination
to imbibe invokes the magic
the aroma swirls
spiriting her away
into the past into the future
she hears the raven's song
and yearns for the feathers
they left her as gifts
outside her window
mementos of the parts of herself
she's forgotten - the deepest parts
- the truest parts
the feathers she collected
she gently gathers
into her own bespoke wing
she uses it to carry her
places far and away
she uses it to soothe
her wandering heart
it is her talisman - her totem
her spirit song

the raven whispers
her deep longing
she sings herself back to life
her wings begin to spread
no longer broken or maimed
she stretches
she ruffles up her midnight down
she begins to sing
her heartache and hopes
she takes another sip of coffee

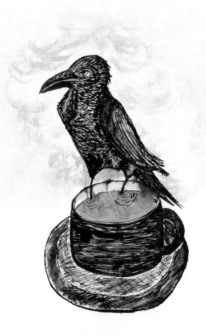

hiking the death trail

the sea speaks
from a distance
a whisper on the wind
calling me out
of my lethargy
what I set out for
hiking the death trail
the one thing killing me
is the thing keeping us alive

but who will care for her?

they say she's too heavy
but her heart
though its seen
many stormy nights
floats lightly on the breeze
the world finds its comfort
upon her cheek
soft - unweathered
let her speak the truth
about her past, the truth
about her future and the truth
about where you came from

she withstands time's
cruel punishment
she endures your pain
her shoulders strong
bearing the heaviness you carry
unhardened and unbroken
unassuming love
and in secret
she will burst into flames
before she sweeps
up the dust and reassembles
herself

gatherer

I collect words
like bones
and sing to them
sometimes they remain
a pile of disembodied
fragments
sometimes magic happens
they come to life
perfect skeletons
dancing in the flames

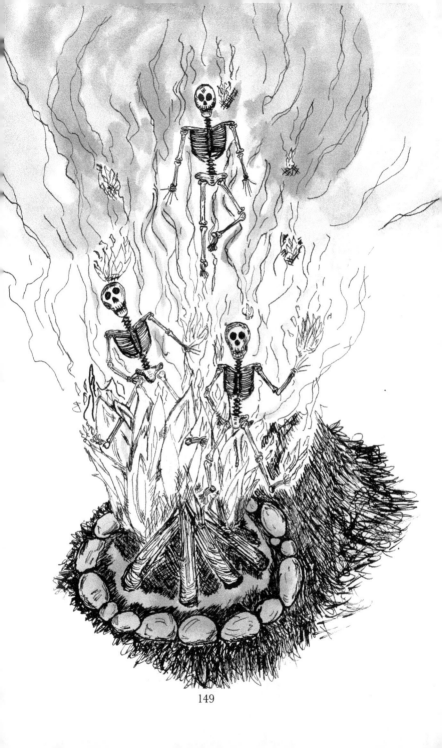

mind state

reality is just another dream
constructed in mind state
if you can see through
to the truth of your dreams
you can more easily see through
the illusion of your reality

gone tomorrow

a beautiful life
lived
an eternal flame
flickers
the energy
moves through
the spirit
lives on

find your wings

in the moments
before I am falling|
I am flying|
what freedom

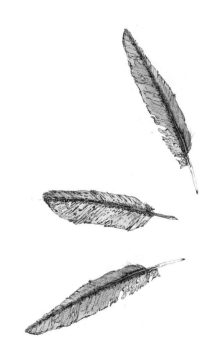

dear, RIP

si belle que tu me fais souffrir
je suis toujours dans ma folie
tu est toujours dans mes rêves
tu me manques

goodbye

an aching deep
a grief that
time stands still for
lungs shudder
then seize
the molecules crystallise
into ice

a heart slows,
can't keep the beat
the only song that
makes any sense
is his voice
carried on the wind
like a whisper

he never does say
goodbye

a tous mes amis qui sont décédé

we've inherited each other
we cast offs, write offs
rejects, drunkards
who find ourselves abandoned
to our own devices
knee deep in our own decay
we'll have a grand tea party
chipped tea cups and
tin can telephones
celebrating our loneliness
we'll tell magnificent stories
eating escargots, ham
and candied sweet potato
first one must bathe in salt
for purification
it will be a mad tea party
and we'll all be mad
madly rushing to our graves
but our selves always catch up by mourning

music

if these words
were music
I'd be dancing
into nothingness
and back again

it's never off key
if you're singing
the truth

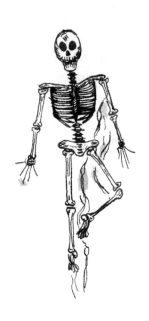

red light, white piano

she's passed by his house before
in the mid-summer heat
when no air flows through
there is no solace of a breeze
he opens all his windows and his front door
to invite some coolness that never arrives
even the dark walls are sweating, stifled

any passer-by becomes an honoured guest
her senses enter without an invitation
perhaps the open door is an invitation
the light is tinted red by a round lampshade
'enter me' it says
straight ahead on a small oak desk
a glass of wine awaits her
above it an oval mirror wall-mounted

he stands watching his reflection
wearing only tight black briefs
taking the stance of a boxer
flexing his biceps in the crimson light
there is a white piano to her left
she enters and begins to play
this being the natural progression
he dances all night to her music
to her song that sets the moon and
wakes the sun and the clouds
and the rain washes her away
he wakes as if from a dream
with her song on his breath

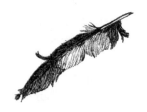

time & relative dimension

if I dive
off the edge
of the precipice
am I choosing lunacy?
the choice is
to never return
rushing headlong
but what awaits me
beyond
is what I fear
myself
I fear my true self
in my external world
my thoughts my feelings
my words my actions
all not suitable
for silent
contemplation
I'm so much bigger
on the inside

a wrinkle

I'm falling again
into space
out of place

all of this magic

all of this magic I've looked for
in his eyes or her smile

I've searched for the magic
in the space between us
but I found it most
growing in me

bread crumbs

this isn't how I planned it
I might have left well enough
alone
I might have let you go
into my wilderness
left you questioning
the best of my intentions
I might have left bread crumbs
and forgotten about them
because I was never lost

mirrors

two selves
separately identical
needs, desires
have more than one face
he sees her
that part of herself
that seeks him out
face to face
mirrors
holy bodies

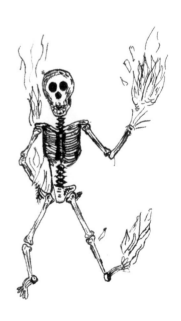

sing your praise

don't let your fear
bind you
don't suffocate
in frozen terror
break free of each mould
you create for yourself
re-invent everyday
the creative act of living
a series of choices you make
release yourself of the shackles
you've built up in your mind
there's a secret place inside
your smile
where you already know
and I'm preaching to the choir
that moment in which you
sing your own praise

beyond wordplay

I heard you
sweetly
a giggle into
the silence
that speaks
beyond wordplay

it's funny though
after all these musings
I have no words left

existing softly
in between
your thoughts
lingering

wake up

wake-up call
when there's a vague
internal restlessness
listen
to the voice
of the wild woman
singing through your bones

perspective

I live in the dark
corners
beyond reason
I see the end
of the rainbow
everyday

maelstrom

I'm racing, idle
through the torrents
of the maelstrom
you bring up in me
the look in your eyes
gives me no reason to hide
I can see tomorrow from here
at the end of the world
you are my home

my secrets

he tastes me
he touches me
he hears me
he sees me
inside everything
every part of me
I do not hide
my secrets
my dark corners
shared, sacred

the sea is my lover

the sea is my lover
when I'm drawn to the ocean
when the moon is high and I
imagine a mystical tryst
under the crashing waves

I have no longing
for another but
for passionate connection
to that wild woman
to goddess
my innermost self

to the undulating
uncontainable
fierce creativity
to wildness
to the untameable

to uncompromising love
the kind no man or woman
could provide
without being swallowed up
sinking into
the depths of my ocean

I know this, so
I do not seek it out
it resides in me

as I long for the unbroken
within me
I fear my own power
my wild creativity
I suppress her
lock her up, hide her away
she's too intimidating
when I let her out

but to survive in this world
she needs to be free
I need to be free
the sea reminds me of this
it calls to her

Isle Poirier

shwaaa haha laashsh shuuh
the smell of this place
takes me home
the crunch of decaying
brown leaves under my feet
the green
the green damp life breathing
the tree stretches out
over the water
Shwaaa haha laashsh shuuh
cradling me
rocking the monster to sleep
as the light waves
lapping up the shore
sing their lullaby
this place breathes
stretching upwards and outwards
it belongs here
everything in this forest belongs
here, I belong here
and the birds know it

wild walked with me

she walked through the fire
the wild walked with her
they danced in the flames
they rose from the ashes as one

la loba

there is a wilderness inside of me
I can barely contain
that I don't want to constrain

it burns fierce - my wild heart
confined to a skeleton
that is bruised and broken

I lick my wounds
I wait, I meditate
dreaming an unbounded existence
wandering savage earth

there is a vast wilderness inside of me
a spirit that will not be tamed or broken
and I burn burn burn
howling at the moon
as it reaches for me

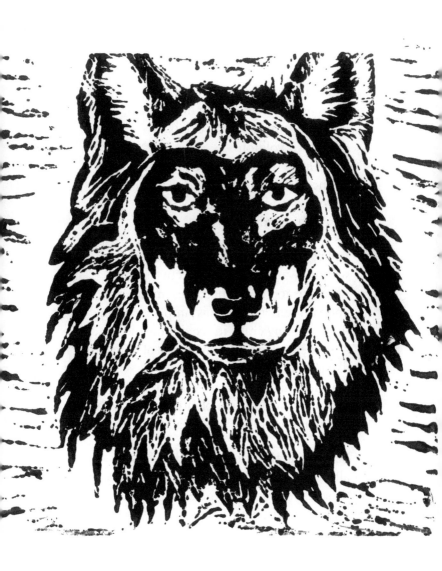

some times

sometimes though, the haze
that engulfs your waking life
choking your inner voice, lifts
of its own volition
sometimes you wake up expecting
all the shit on those ever-growing lists
of to do's and not enough's
to weigh you down

you've prepared for the worst when
without warning, all perspective shifts
what was too heavy becomes immaterial
and you remember life is simply beautiful
there is a tiny crack in fixed time and space
a moment of clarity, a memory of tomorrow
like looking out at the ocean
your feet dig deep into the sand, the skyline
completely cloud-free blending into the horizon
and you remember what really matters

because all the knocks and the blows
all the failures and the triumphs aren't you
these experiences you give weight to
and carry wherever you go
helped guide you here
        - like backseat drivers
to this breath of clarity where

everything comes into balance

and when you look out of yourself
wherever it is you happen to be when
you open your eyes to beauty in all things
you'll know this moment can sustain you
if you arrive with it and continue to
arrive in each following moment
you allow that single breath to guide
your next

it is there to remind you
of what is real and true, and to let go
of what binds you to the ache of the past
or the anxiety of the future
and the next time you're lost
in the jungle you can recall
the ebb and flow of the ocean and
when you breathe, you breathe what is true

little joys

we were talking
about suffering
about how the mind runs
about habitual pain
I long for health
but when that longing disappoints
I can choose despair or I can
choose grace
I open myself to the little joys
why would I choose to suffer
what I cannot escape?

we don't suffer because we hurt
but because we want not to
disease - physical pain
emotional turmoil - financial strain
we despair, we fear, we resist
we long for ease

we hold a magnifying glass
to that which we want not to see
and our joy is diminished
no pleasant experience
is ever enough
it could always be more, better, bigger, easier

the moment is heavy
with what we bring to it
we cannot see things as they are
we cannot accept what
we cannot change

we cannot change
this moment
so we judge it
we quantify it
unpleasant, avoid
pleasant, hold fast

then joy evades us
when we have it
we fear losing it
we want more, better, bigger, easier
we hold on tight
we lose sight
chasing our own tails

so I try
I recognise it in myself
I choose joy
I invite grace
I suffer less
and find love in its place

(*First published on Elephant Journal June 2017*)

öm

ever
and ever
and ever
will I fall
      and climb
fall
      and fly
ever
will I fade
disperse into
      particles
moving
      chaotically
and in
      unison
creating, sustaining, destroying
being
created, sustained, destroyed
      employed
      idle
in idleness I am
never stasis
always creating
      being created
      thinking
      feeling
repose

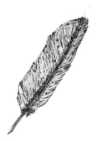

love is

love is
the feeling
you have
when you
look
your cat
in the eyes
and she softly
blinks

the only way through is in

floating in the ink river
through a tunnel
I enter a cave
immersed
in the darkness
in the black

he reaches out to me
raises me up
"how do I get above ground
to the forest
to the light"
I ask

his eyes
like burning coals
shine, smiling
"when you see truly
in the dark
you will not need
the light"

the dampness
of the cave walls
glistens like stars
in the night sky

inhale
exhale
I am weightless
I am stardust
among the stars

shadow wolf

he's my shadow
he's my light
his unselfish love
is my constant
reminder
to keep searching
through the dark
to keep the flame
burning
in my heart

what feels right

what feels right
when you scoop me up
when you hold me in
when our eyes meet
they lock into each other
the connecting pieces
to a puzzle we didn't know
existed

longtime now

when I look into your eyes
a deep urge to smile
stirs and leaps up
from the softness below
in between my ribs
where my light is
even when I think I hate you
even in a fit of rage
even after all these years
I look into you and
all the bullshit seems
so small compared to
the depth of my feeling
that's how I know
I just love you

promises, promises

the promise of the sun
a warm embrace is lost
to the biting winds
blowing a winter gale
my bones ache
the sun is a liar
the moon never lies
I live for the truth
and love by the moon

time

I wasn't looking
to find
that which I seek
but as it happens
so it goes
and I flow
with it riding
the waves curling
up through me
you see
that game we all play
with time
stop
too fast
too slow
too much
not enough
grounds for control
to see clearly within
the construct of time
herein lies the truth
we are now
sans prologue
epilogue

but let the narrative
begin
at the start
progressing through
every momentous existence
unlike the book
time has no end

perfection

perfection
isn't an achievement
isn't striving
isn't out there

perfection
is the moment
is now
is you
it is the whole
complete
chaotic
mess

in the end

brief encounters
skipping stones
and scattered bones
words fall short
of sense and worlds
write it out anyway
don't be afraid to leave
footprints in the sand
however small
your feet are
they all get washed away
in the end

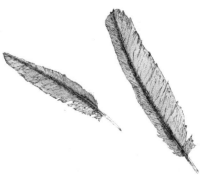

what it is to be free

row on row
of stagnancy set in stone
erect for me a tree
remember me now
as I was before
send me then
in all directions
where I may whisper
and dance through the leaves
that I may experience
what it is to be free

stardust

words pull at my hair
wild under the moon
whisper frantic alight
they guide my journey
through the dark
becoming stardust
by the morn

inevitable

avoiding the inevitable
all things must end
just as all things have begun

epilogue

November 7, 2016

so long, my love
to the man
in the hat
who sang the words
all the right words
if anything was ever
worth much at all
it was his words
that created the
world
I inhabited so naturally
where everywhere else
I was displaced
I am a character he
created
I belong to his words
I belong to his song
and when he says, so long
my love, carry on
we're all so much bigger on the inside
see the light seeping through

Acknowledgements

Thank you.

My sincerest gratitude to Yasmin Gray (Hamid), Chantelle Malone and Dad for your invaluable help and insights through the production of this collection from editing to layout and design.

To my Canadian and Australian family, for your constant love & support. And for your encouragement to keep creating through the trials of being chronically ill.

To my lyme community, for sharing in my heartbreaks and triumphs. Your perseverance inspires me.

To Nigel Gray for your guidance and encouragement over the years.

To my dear friends & early readers for your enthusiasm.

To my husband, Sandy, for being a patron of the arts.

To Cohen, for being my constant.

About the Author

Andrea Sheldon is a writer and artist whose work orbits themes of chronic illness, solitude, melancholia, womanhood, spirituality, mysticism, and mythos. Andrea was born in Montreal, Canada and is currently based in Dongara, Australia with her husband, Sandy, and their blue cattle dog named Cohen. When she isn't tucked away in a room of her own absorbed in her latest project, you can find her eating plants and walking Cohen on the beach. You can find fragments of her at www.andreasheldon.org.

CPSIA information can be obtained
at www.ICGtesting.com
Printed in the USA
BVHW070757020119
536776BV00019B/3850/P